This book is dedicated
to the joy-filled memory of my father,
who loved life, and lived love

# THE GIFT OF
# YEARS

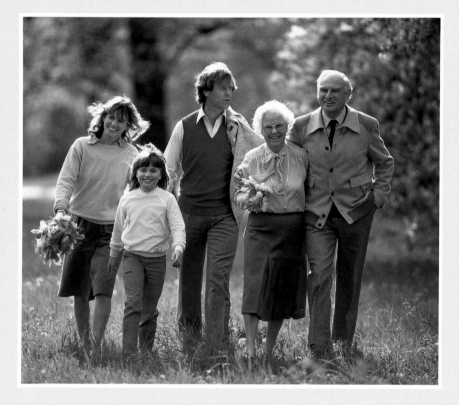

Written and compiled by Marion Stroud

INSPIRATIONAL PRESS

NEW YORK

Published in 1991 by
Inspirational Press
A division of LDAP, Inc.
386 Park Avenue South
Suite 1913
New York, NY  10016

Inspirational Press is a registered trademark of LDAP, Inc.

Published by arrangement with Lion Publishing plc, Oxford,
England, and Lion Publishing Corporation, Batavia, Illinois.

ISBN: 0-88486-046-9

Printed In Italy

### Acknowledgments

The photographs in this book are reproduced by permission of the following
photographers and organizations:
Alan Bedding: 'Thank you'.
Sonia Halliday Photographs/Sister Daniel: 'Changing scenes', 'Peace in the pain', 'True
greatness'; Jane Taylor: 'The letter'.
Lion Publishing/David Alexander: 'The good life' (centre), 'On the other side'.
Picturepoint: 'The grand adventure', 'Something beautiful'.
Jean-Luc Ray: 'Across the years' (left-hand page).
Doug Sewell: 'Never alone'.
Tony Stone: 'The gift of years', 'A wider family', 'Across the years (right-hand page),
'What is a grandmother?'.
Vision International: 'Life is for living' (left-hand page), 'Dark days'.
All remaining photographs by ZEFA.

Bible quotations as follows: James 1:17 ('Changing scenes'), Philippians 1:6 ('Something
beautiful'), Romans 8:28 ('Peace in the pain'), Hebrews 13:5,6 ('All our care'), John 11:25,
Revelation 21:3,4, 1 Corinthians 15:54-57 ('On the other side') from *Holy Bible, New
International Version,* copyright 1978 New York International Bible Society; Joshua
14:11,12 ('Take the high road') from *Good News Bible,* copyright 1966, 1971 and 1976
American Bible Society, published by Bible Societies/Collins; Isaiah 46:3,4 ('Something
beautiful') from *The Living Bible,* copyright 1971 Tyndale House Publishers.

Other copyright material as follows: 'The good life' from *The Time of Your Life* by Herb
and Mary Montgomery, Winston Press; 'The grand adventure' from *The Adventure of
Living* by Paul Tournier, reprinted by permission of Highland Books; extract from
'Stopping by Woods on a Snowy Evening' by Robert Frost, from *The Poems of Robert
Frost* edited by Edward Connery Lathem, reprinted by permission of Jonathan Cape
Ltd and Holt, Rinehart and Winston; extract by Gigi Tchividjian under 'Something
beautiful' from *A Woman's Search for Serenity,* reprinted by permission of Fleming
H. Revell Company; extracts by David Watson under 'A wider family' from *In Search of
God,* a Falcon Books publication, reprinted by permission of Kingsway Publications Ltd
and 'On the other side' from *Through the Year with David Watson* © 1982 by Jean Watson,
reprinted by permission of Hodder and Stoughton Ltd; 'Thank you, God, that it's here'
from *Hold Me Up a Little Longer, Lord* by Marjorie Holmes, copyright © 1977 by Marjorie
Holmes Mighell, reprinted by permission of Doubleday and Company, Inc. and
Hodder and Stoughton Ltd *(Lord, Let Me Love);* 'There's so much of me, in me, Lord',
first published in the Australian magazine *Christian Woman;* 'The letter' by Doris Haase,
reprinted by permission from *Daily Guideposts, 1979,* copyright © 1978 by Guideposts
Associates, Inc., New York; 'I have been giving thought, Lord' from *You have a minute,
Lord?* by David Kossoff, reprinted by permission of Robson Books Ltd.

Youth and age are not dates in time, but states of mind.
Our duty is not to add years to our lives,
but to add life to our years. . .
Time may wrinkle the skin, but worry, doubt, hate
and the loss of ideals wrinkle the soul.
Fears, not years, bow the head. . .
Whether we are seventy or seventeen,
a sense of the wonder of life keeps us young.

*Myron J. Taylor*

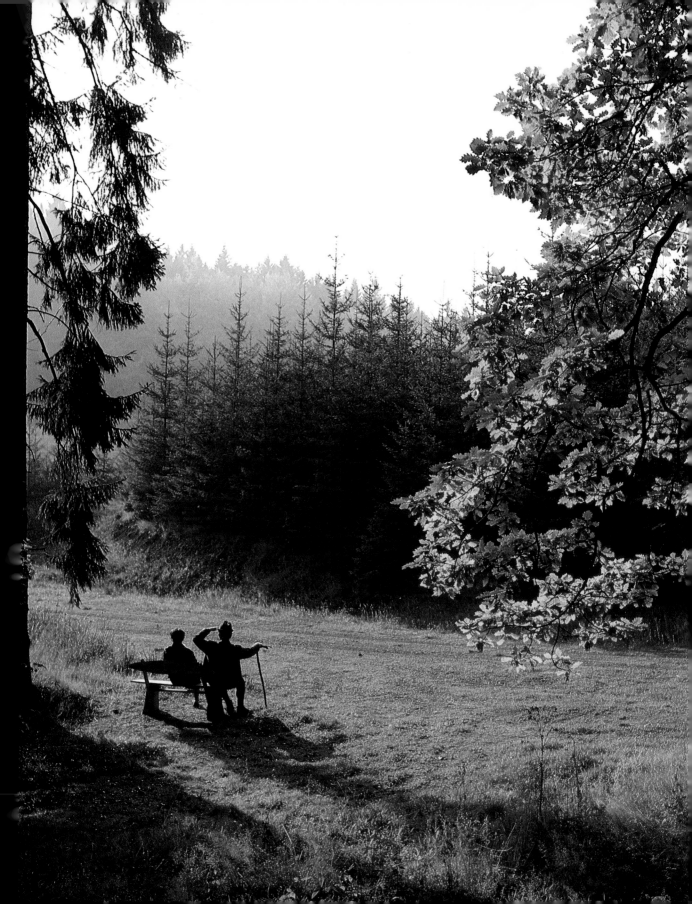

# THE OAK

Live thy life
Young and old
Like yon oak,
Bright in Spring,
Living gold;

Summer – rich
Then; and then
Autumn – changed,
Soberer-hued,
Gold again.

All his leaves
·Fall'n at length
Look, he stands
Trunk and bough
Naked strength.

*Alfred Tennyson*

# THE GIFT OF YEARS

The gift of years is an invisible package that must be opened and enjoyed one day at a time. We cannot buy it, sell it or hoard it as a hedge against the time when we are confronted with a certain shortage of future.

The gift of years contains freedom from old ties but responsibility for new ones. It holds joy and pain, laughter and tears, success and defeat, triumph and disaster.

Within its wrappings we may discover the next-but-one generation. We struggle to become supportive but non-interfering in-laws; loving grandparents, great-aunts or uncles; wise counsellors or receptive counsellees. We learn to be people who are willing to receive as well as to share; to hold out the experience we have gained over the years in an open hand so that it can be accepted or rejected at will.

The gift of years may hold bodily weakness and limitations but it can also contain increased spiritual strength and effectiveness.

It is a free gift that cannot be earned nor must we take it for granted, for it is not presented to all equally.

The gift of years must simply be received with thanksgiving, for it is the gift of life itself.

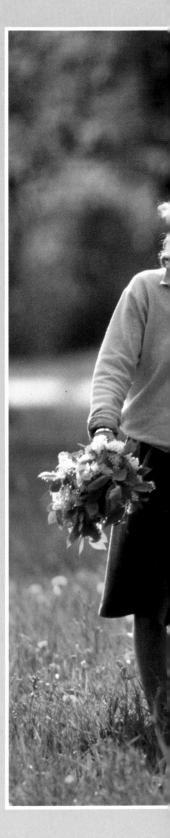

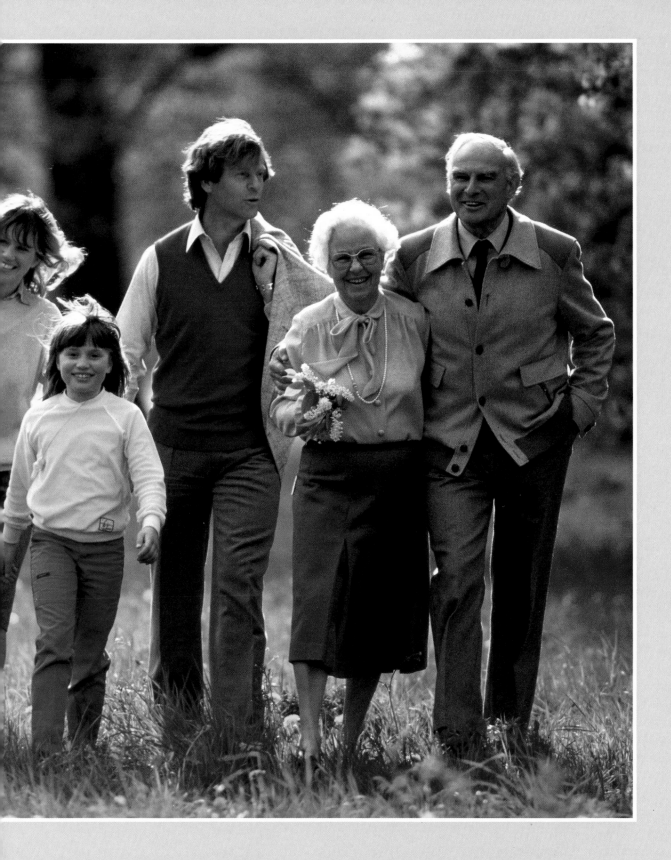

# THE GOOD LIFE

Many of us spend time believing that the 'good life' is going to begin some time in the future. It's going to be great when we've got enough money, when we meet someone who truly understands us, when we have our own business, when we retire. But life doesn't begin in the future. Right now is the time of our life! When we realize this, the hours we have take on greater worth. We see clearly that using our time well is important because each minute is a miracle that cannot be repeated.

   Making the most of every moment is no accident. Those who live life to the full do so with design and purpose. They realize the value of time and see the world as a place of wonder and new possibilities.

*Herb and Mary Montgomery*

If you want to do something, do it today. Say sorry, show someone you love them *now*. If you have had a row, make it up. Don't waste time.

*Daphne Hamilton Fairley*

The good life is a *process*, not a state of being. It is a direction, not a destination.

*Carl Rogers*

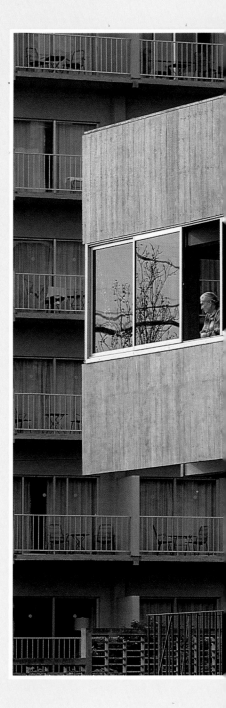

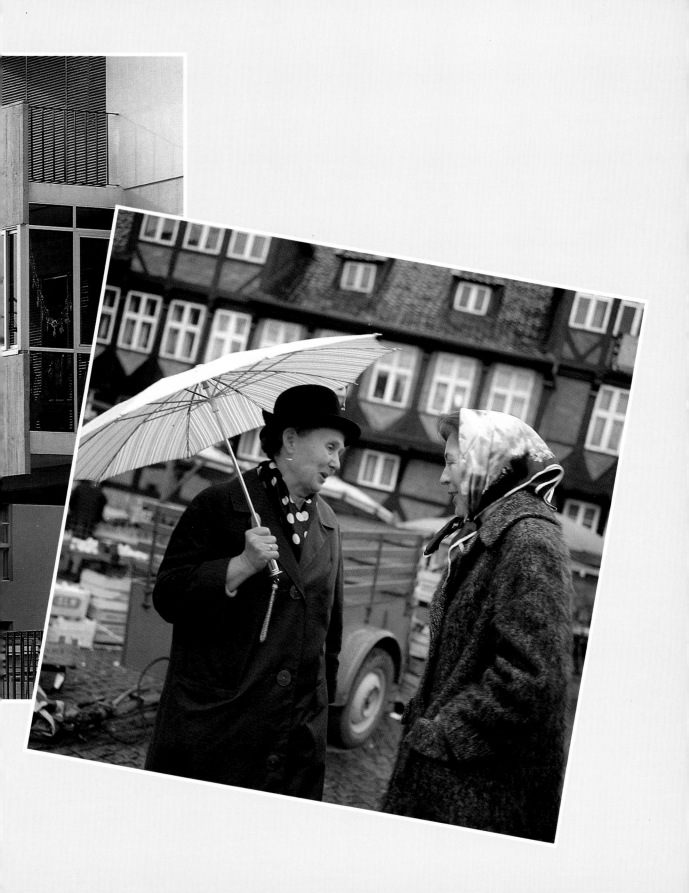

# THE GRAND ADVENTURE

At any moment an unsatisfying life may become once more a grand adventure if we will surrender it to God. . .He is the very source of life, a source that is always new. He brings one adventure to an end, only to open another to us. He is tireless and inexhaustible. With him we must be ready for anything.

The adventure of faith is exciting, difficult and exacting, but full of poetry, of new discoveries, of fresh turns and sudden surprises.

The God of the Bible is the God who acts. He is the God who commits himself in every man's life. He does not interest himself only in man's religious life but in his whole life. . .in his occupation – and he turns that occupation into a veritable adventure.

*Paul Tournier*

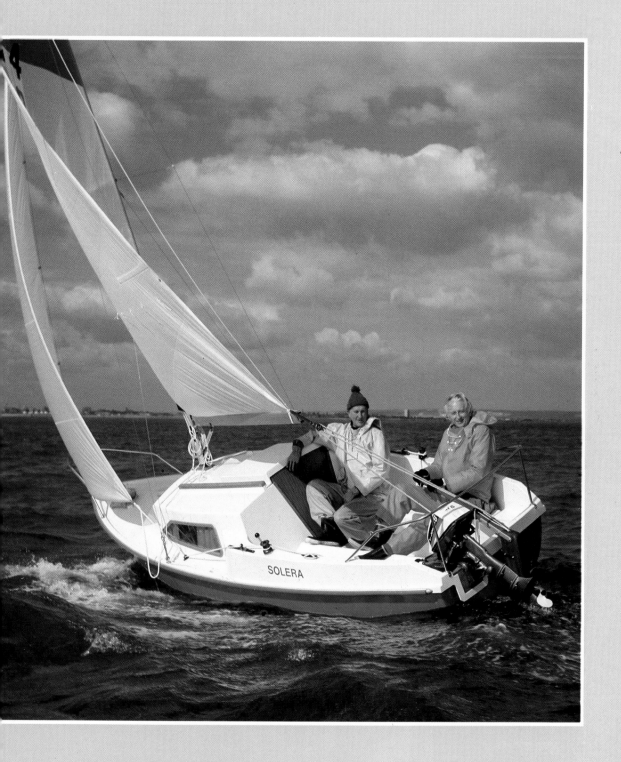

# CHANGING SCENES

'Every good. . .gift is from above, coming. . .from the Father. . .who does not change.'

*James: from the New Testament*

'Change is one of the few things in life that is certain,' he said, 'since change and growth are two sides of the same coin. Every period of change, whether it is from childhood to adult life, singleness to marriage, middle life to old age, requires some degree of giving up and letting go. So growth can either be a painful or a rewarding experience. It all depends whether we fight it or accept it. Remember, hands which are

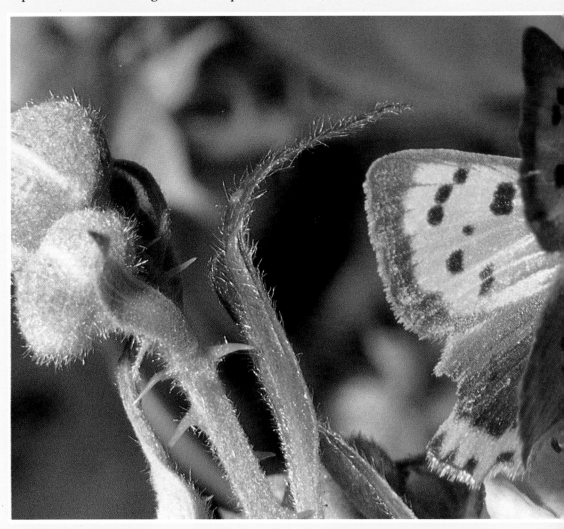

grimly clutching onto the past, are totally unable to grasp hold of the present and the future.'

'Clutching onto the past or grasping the present' – it's so easy to do the first, Lord. To cling resolutely to the happiness, achievements and people in my past, while refusing to see that it is part of life's pattern that my relationships, life-style and goals should change with the years, as well as my appearance.

Thank you that you deal so gently with me, Lord. Remind me often that every day is a gift from you, to be tasted and savoured as if life itself has just begun, and that you intend me to develop one day and one year at a time, taking with me into the future the best of every stage experienced thus far.

The future sometimes looks a little frightening, Lord. Thank you that there is no pathway I need tread without your company. And thank you, Father, that in all the changing scenes of life one thing is certain: you are the same yesterday, today and for ever.

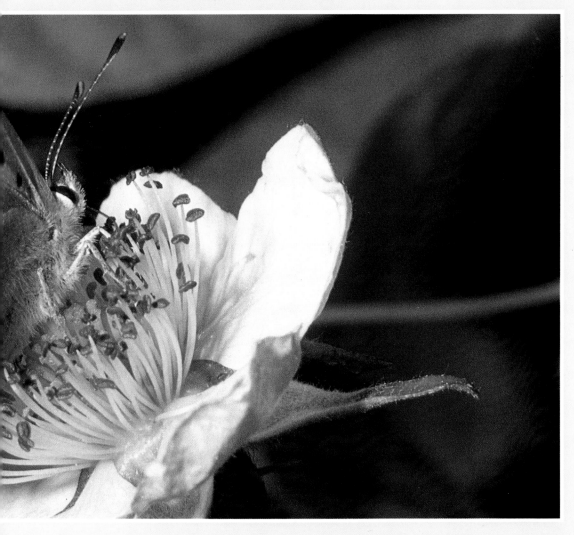

# TAKE THE HIGH ROAD

*'Caleb. . .said. . ."Look at me!. . .I am still strong enough for war or for anything else. Now then, give me the hill-country that the Lord promised me on that day when my men and I reported. We told you then that. . .giants. . .were there in large walled cities. . .the Lord will be with me, and I will drive them out."'*

The Book of Joshua

Is this what they call the 'mid-life crisis', Lord? This feeling that life must surely have more to offer than I have experienced so far, coupled with a strange reluctance to go out and get involved with it? One half of me refuses to accept that challenge and excitement are the prerogative of the young (after all, Lord, Caleb was eighty when he picked the toughest part of the Promised Land for his inheritance!), and the other half whispers, 'Slow down a bit! It's time that someone else took on the tough jobs. You have done your share; enjoy life, relax a little.'

It's a tempting thought, Lord! And yet my better self knows that I could never be really satisfied with the soft option. That your call is not for a few years but for life. And that the mountain climbed in your company is infinitely preferable to the self-chosen easy road, which I would have to walk alone.

So re-fire me, Lord. Give me a fresh vision of where I am going, and why. Enable me to see what your plan is for this stage of my life, and help me to give all I've got in the doing of it. If you will lead me on, then surely I will 'strive with things impossible, and get the better of them'.

The woods are lovely, dark and deep,
But I have promises to keep,
And miles to go before I sleep.

*Robert Frost*

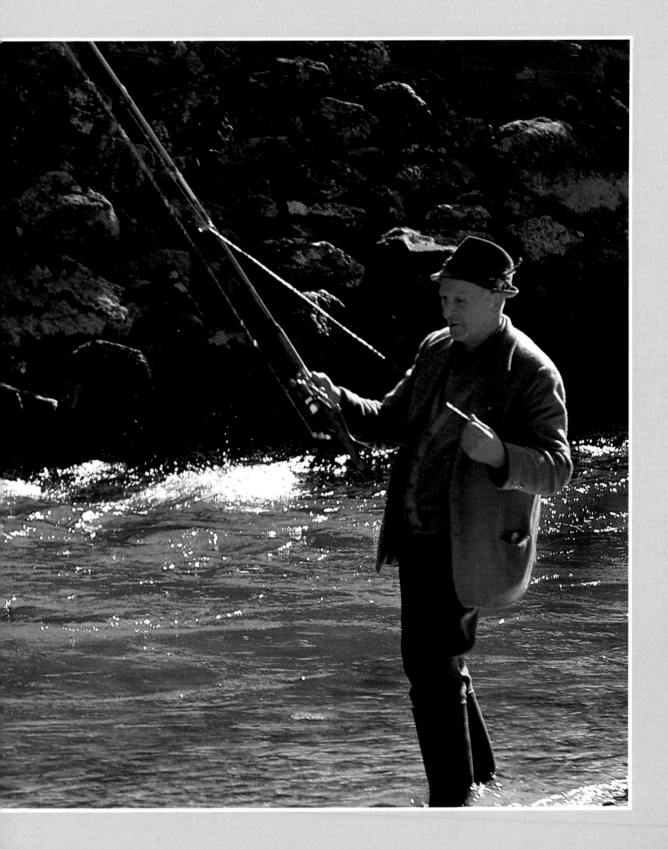

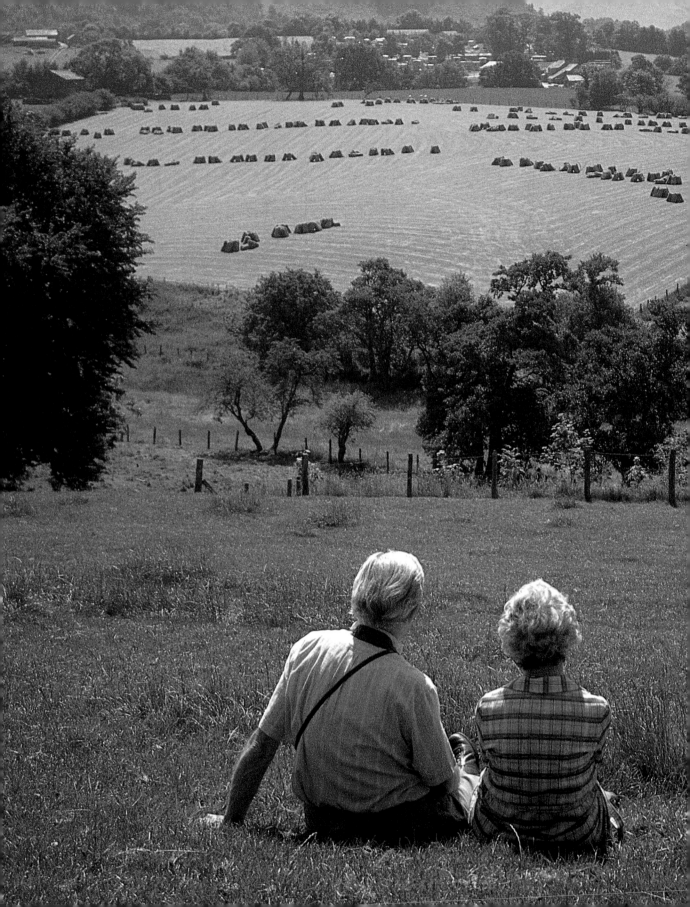

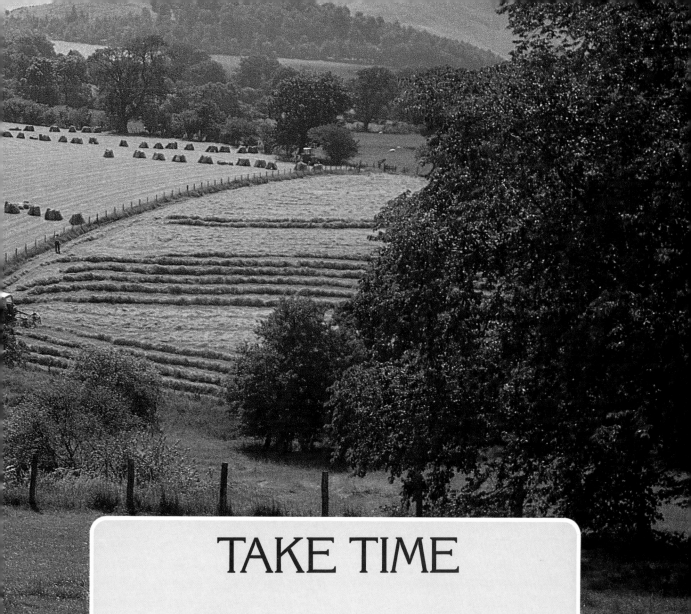

# TAKE TIME

Take time to work – it is the price of success.
Take time to think – it is the source of power.
Take time to play – it is the secret of perpetual youth.
Take time to read – it is the fountain of wisdom.
Take time to be friendly – it is a road to happiness.
Take time to dream – it is hitching your wagon to a star.
Take time to love and be loved – it is the privilege of redeemed people.
Take time to look around – it is too short a day to be selfish.
Take time to laugh – it is the music of the soul.
Take time for God – it is life's only lasting investment.

*Anon*

# THE FRIEND OF SILENCE

We need to find God, and he cannot be found in noise and restlessness. God is the friend of silence. See how nature – trees, flowers, grass – grow in silence; see how the stars, the moon and sun, how they move in silence. . .The more we receive in silent prayer, the more we can give in our active life. . .The essential thing is not what we say, but what God says to us. . .words which do not give the light of Christ increase the darkness.

*Mother Teresa*

Come now. . .flee for a little while from your tasks; hide yourself for a little space from the turmoil of your thoughts. Come, cast aside your burdensome care and your laborious pursuits. For a little while give your time to God and rest in him. . .shut out all things save God, and whatever may aid you in seeking God; and having barred the door of your chamber, seek him.

*Anselm of Canterbury*

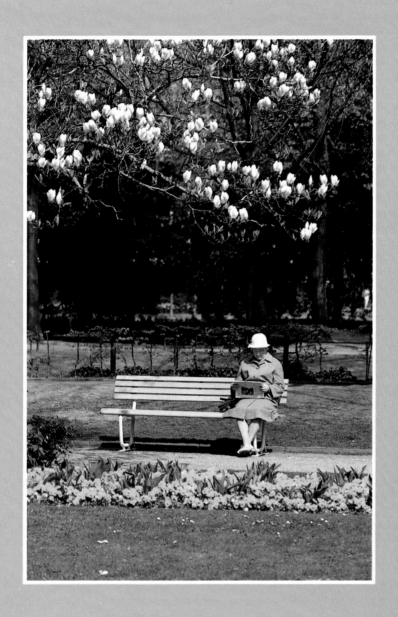

# LIFE IS FOR LIVING

There is no experience from which you can't learn something. When you stop learning, you stop living in any vital and meaningful sense. And the purpose of life, after all, is to live it, to taste experience to the utmost, to reach out eagerly and without fear for newer and richer experience.

*Eleanor Roosevelt*

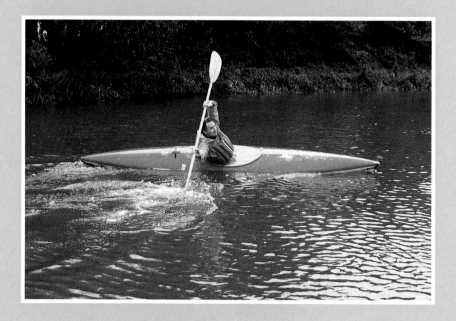

Many times the only way we can find out what is possible is by finding out what is not possible – in other words, by making a mistake.

*Nelson Boswell*

The man who never made a mistake never made anything.

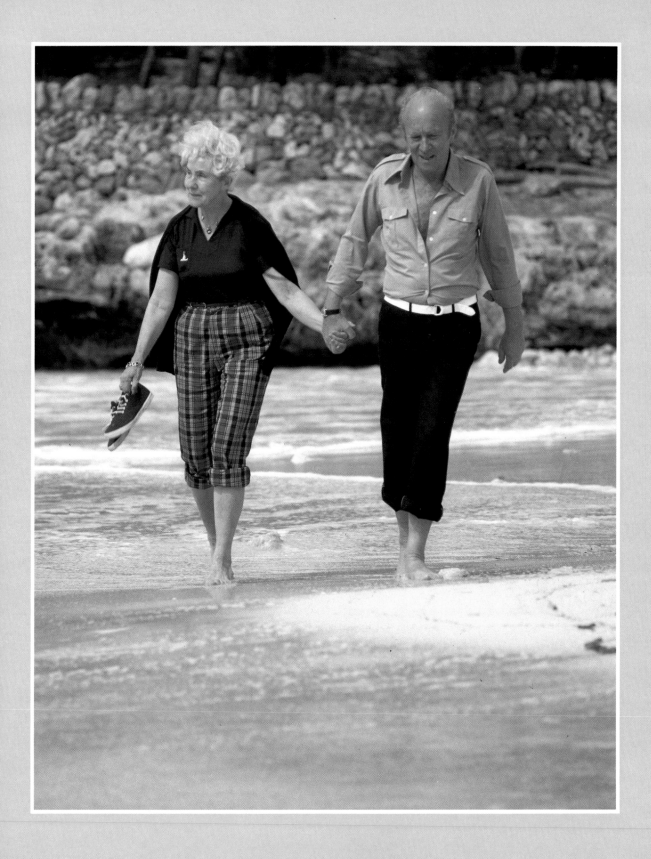

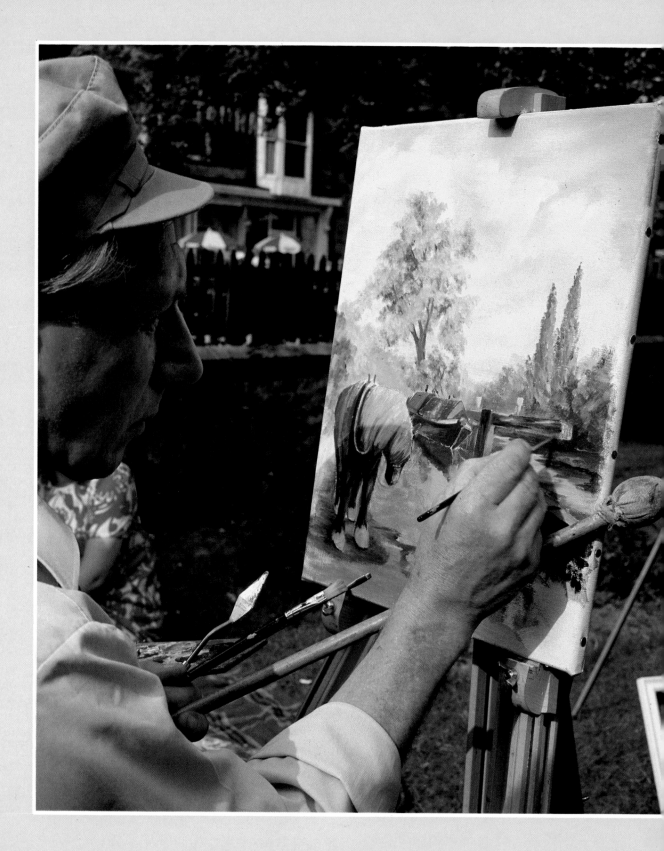

# SOMETHING BEAUTIFUL

*'The Lord will perfect that which concerns me. . .'*

The Book of Psalms

*'He who began a good work in you will carry it on to completion. . .'*

Paul: from the New Testament


'The story is told of an old Italian artist who had lost some of his skill. One evening he sat discouraged before a painting he had just completed. He noticed that he had lost some of his touch. The canvas didn't burst with life as once it did, and he went sadly to bed.

'Later his son, also an artist, came to examine his father's work, and he, too, noticed the lack. Taking the palette, he worked far into the night, adding a little touch here, a smudge there, a little colour here, a shadow there. He worked until the picture fulfilled his father's vision.

'Morning came, and when the father entered the studio, he stood in utter delight before his perfect canvas and exclaimed, "Why, I have wrought better than I knew!"

'One day, we too will look upon the canvas of our lives, and because of the touch of Jesus on it. . .we too will fulfill God the Father's vision.' We will discover that his loving skill has transformed the blots and blemishes into things of beauty. And the Father will look, not on our work, but on what Jesus has accomplished, and will see the picture perfected.

*Adapted from Gigi Tchividjian*


Something beautiful, something good,
All my confusion He understood.
All I had to offer Him
Was brokenness and strife,
But He made something beautiful of my life.

*William J. Gaither*

# NEVER ALONE

*'Listen to me. . .I have created you and cared for you since you were born.
I will be your God through all your life-time, yes, even when your hair is
white with age. I made you and I will care for you. I will carry you along
and be your Saviour.'*

The Book of Isaiah

One night a man had a dream. He dreamed he was walking along
the beach with the Lord. Across the sky flashed scenes from his life.
Each scene, he noticed, began with two sets of footprints in the
sand: one belonging to him, and the other to the Lord.

When the last scene of his life flashed before him, he looked back
at the footprints in the sand. He noticed that at times along the path
of his life, the pattern altered, so that there was only one set of
footprints. He also noticed that it happened at the very lowest and
saddest times in his life. This really troubled him and he questioned
the Lord about it.

'Lord, you said that once I decided to follow you, you'd walk with
me all the way. But I've noticed that during the most troublesome
times in my life, there is only one set of footprints. I don't
understand why, when I needed you most, you would leave me.'

The Lord replied, 'My son, my precious child, I love you and
I would never leave you. During your time of trial and suffering,
when you see only one set of footprints, it was then that I carried
you.'

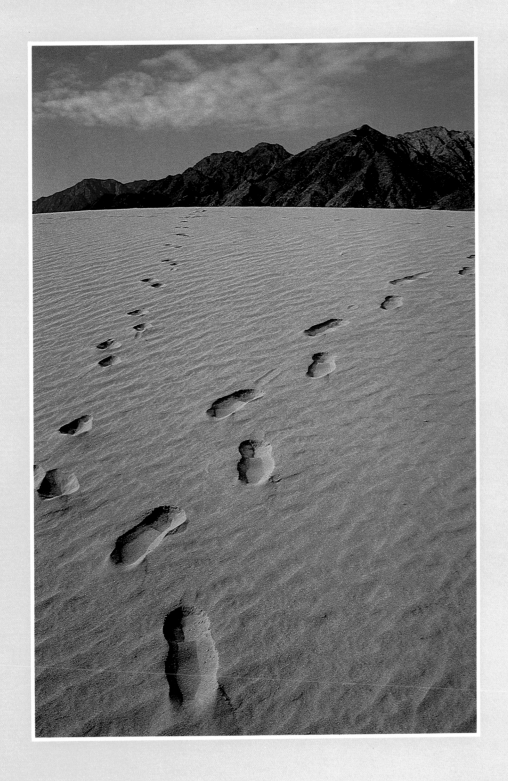

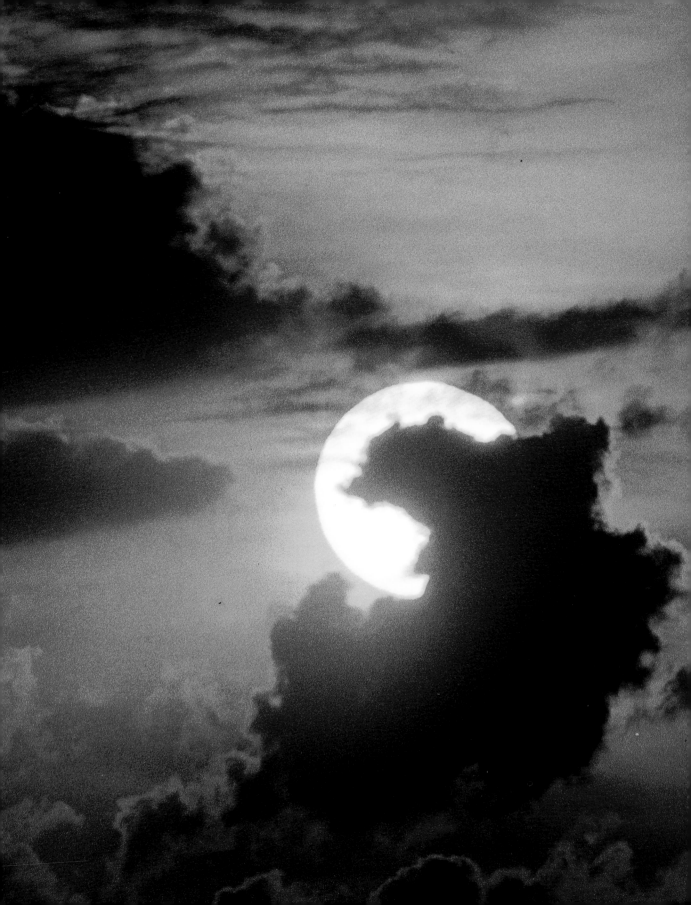

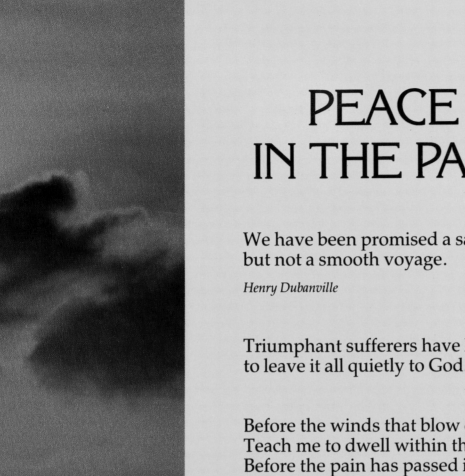

# PEACE
# IN THE PAIN

We have been promised a safe arrival
but not a smooth voyage.

*Henry Dubanville*

Triumphant sufferers have learned
to leave it all quietly to God.

Before the winds that blow do cease,
Teach me to dwell within thy calm;
Before the pain has passed in peace,
Give me, my God, to sing a psalm;
Let me not lose the chance to prove
The fulness of enabling love.

*Amy Carmichael*

*We know that in all things God works
for the good of those who love him.*

Paul: from the New Testament

# DARK DAYS

To protect them from pain. Surely this is what every mother longs to do. To shield them from the hurts, the problems and the pressures of life. To gather them up in my arms as once I could do, and soothe their tears with a kiss, a cuddle and a gentle word.

But life is not like that any more. Although I sometimes pray 'Lord, let me take it for them – I can bear it, let them go free', I know that this is not God's way. His loving dealings with us involve correction, testing and dark days, as well as laughter, joy and sunlit pathways. And the one without the other would produce a lop-sided character, weak and underdeveloped in young and old alike.

So I cannot protect them from pain. I can only stand there with them in it – available but not intrusive, loving but not smothering, watchful but not inquisitive. And I can pray. Not for an easy journey, but for the stout shoes of faith and courage and love, which will enable them to tread the roughest path in safety.

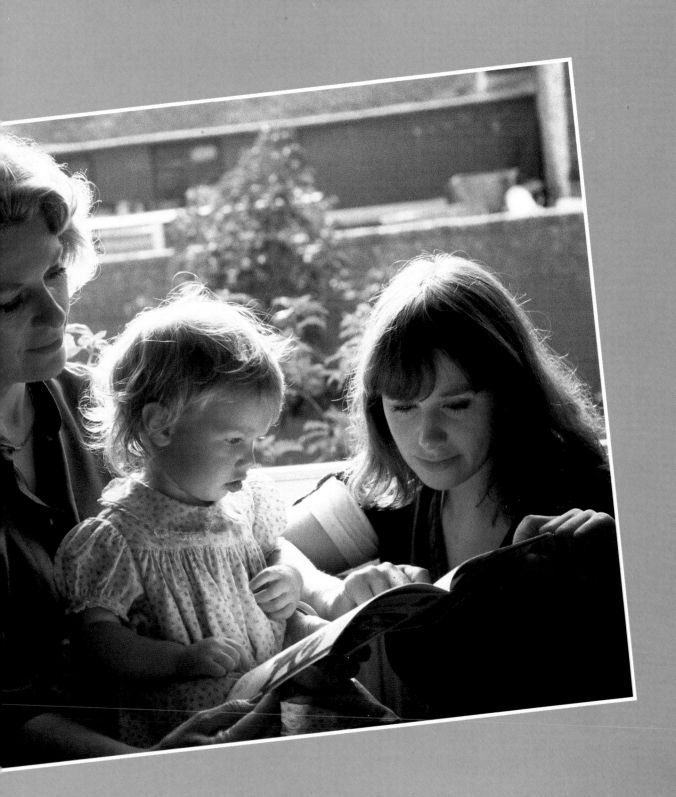

# A WIDER FAMILY

*'If I become bitter and resentful in my suffering, I shall still have my suffering but on top of that, I have to contend with my bitterness and resentment as well; and this may be even worse than my initial suffering. . .If in my suffering I open my heart to the love and peace and friendship of Jesus Christ, then this will wonderfully transform the entire situation.'*

David Watson

I thought that I had come to terms with it, Lord. That the pain was over, and that I had learned to think of us as a 'child-free' rather than a 'childless' couple. To concentrate on the good part of being a twosome rather than a family, and to offer you the ache in my heart and the emptiness in my arms whenever I peeped admiringly into a pram, or was caught in conversation near the school gates.

But today it is back, washed in on a tidal wave of other people's family joy. Why did I have to meet them all in one short hour's shopping? Jenny – a grandmother by Christmas, she says; Margaret, trying on that ridiculous hat for her son's wedding; and Christine, full of her coming visit to her daughter's family on the other side of the world. And while I smiled and congratulated them one by one, my heart cried out all over again, Why, God, why? Why have we been excluded from this beautiful and exclusive club called 'Parenthood'?

For it isn't just me, you know, Lord! My husband feels it too. Other men have the exploits of their children and grandchildren with which to enliven their conversation and brighten their leisure hours. They may grumble about the expense and the anxiety, but not for a moment would they exchange their situation for his, however much they might appear to envy him his freedom.

Please help me, Lord. Deal with the hurt, the sense of something missing and that corroding self-pity that sears my heart as painfully as any branding iron. And please reassure me – that there will be someone, somewhere, who will welcome my visits when I am old.

I know that I need to focus on the good things that have enriched our life: the freedom to travel and to enjoy our friends and wider family; the extra time that we have been able to give to nephews and nieces who talk to us with a frankness that would amaze their parents. And the students, who have occupied our spare bedroom and filled the kitchen with smells of exotic cooking – widening our horizons with their varieties of culture and belief. Children of our own we may have lacked. . .but never love. Love of family, love of friends, and most constant of all, your love. For that priceless gift which brightens the future, and gently dispels the darkness of today, I thank you, Lord.

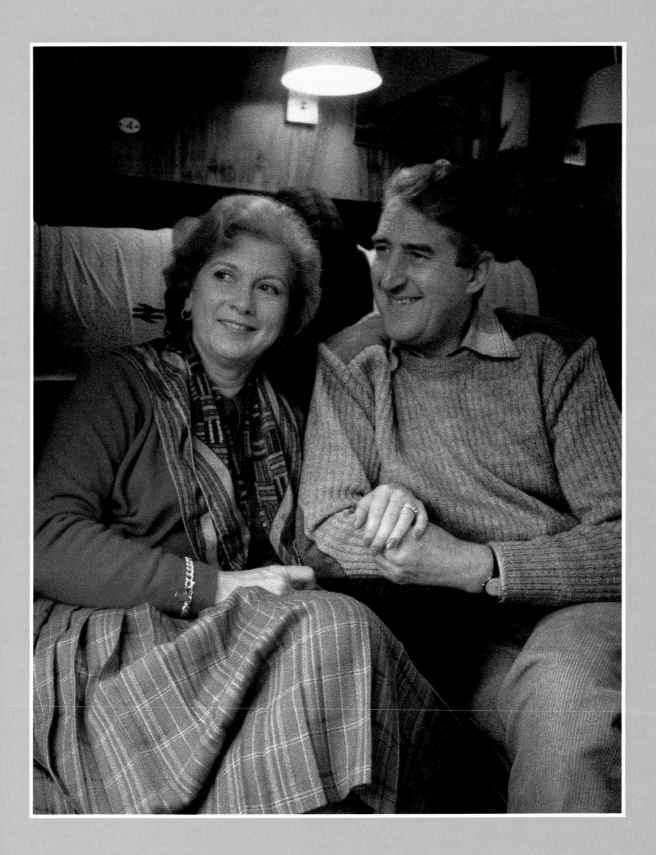

# ACROSS THE YEARS

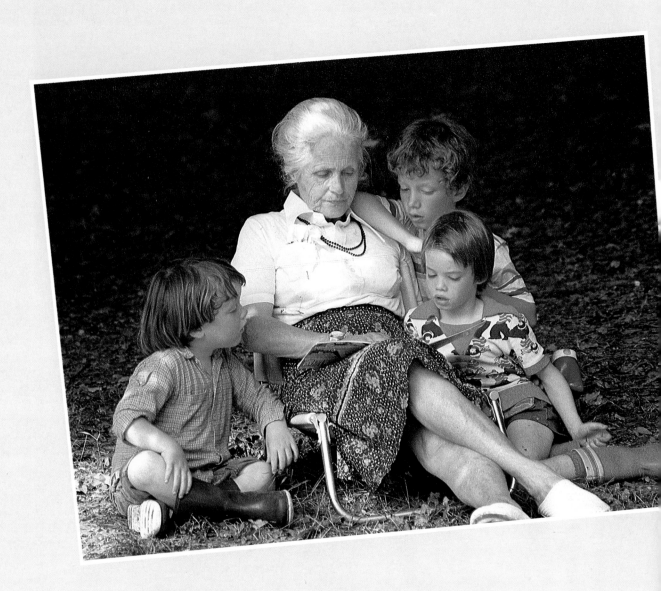

Grandparents need grandchildren to keep the changing
world alive for them. And grandchildren need grandparents
to help them know who they are and to give them a sense of
human experience in a world they cannot know.

*Margaret Mead*

A grandfather has the wisdom of long experience and the love of an understanding heart. He is more interested in the happiness of his children and grandchildren than anything else in the world. He can reminisce with them and share their dreams with interest and enthusiasm. He is the head of a family that loves him and looks up to him with respect and pride. He is a wonderful man to know and love.

*Dean Walley*

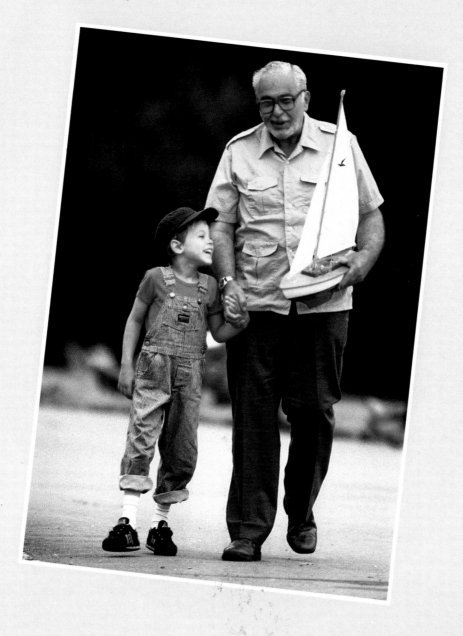

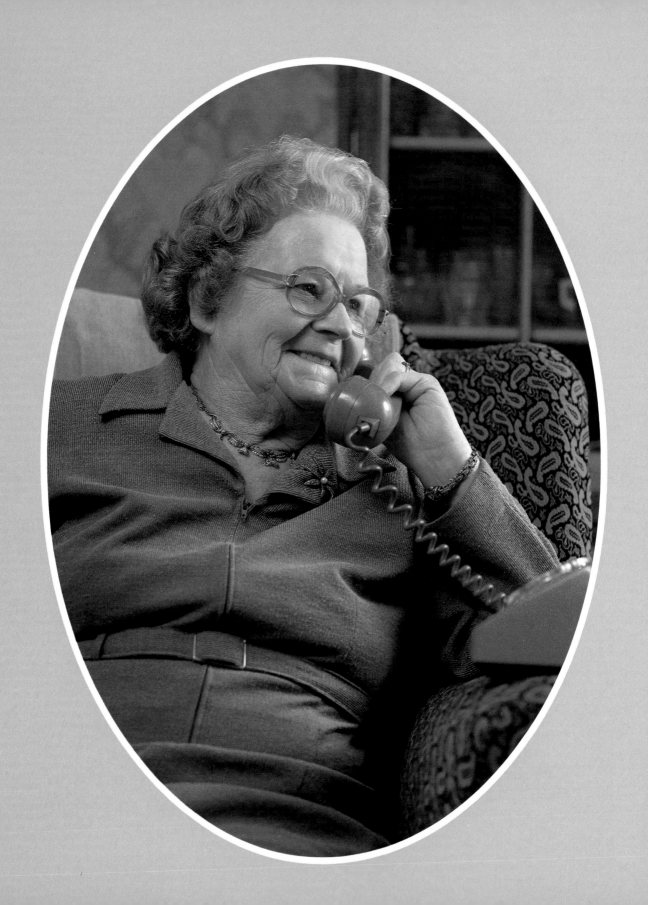

# FIRST GRANDCHILD

Thank you, God, that it's here, our
first grandchild!

I hang up the telephone, rejoicing.
I gaze out the window, dazzled and
awed. 'Just a few moments ago,' he
said. 'A beautiful little girl.'

She arrived with the sunrise, Lord.
The heavens are pink with your glory.
Radiance streams across the world.

The very trees lift up their branches as
if in welcome, as if to receive her. And
I want to fling out my arms, too, in joy
and gratefulness and welcome.

My arms and my heart hold her up to
you for blessing.

Oh, Lord, thank you for her and bless
her, this little new life that is
beginning its first day.

*Marjorie Holmes*

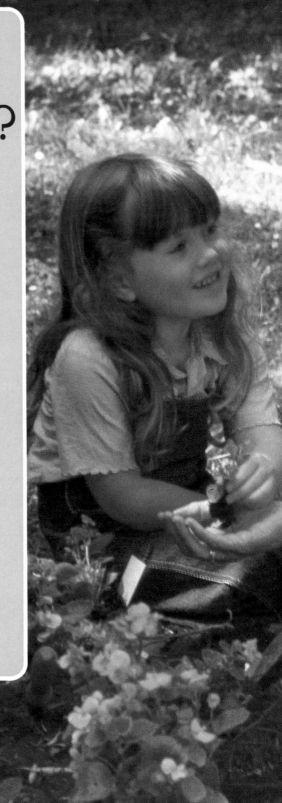

# WHAT IS A GRANDMOTHER?

'A grandmother is a lady who has no children of her own. She likes other people's little girls and boys.

'Grandmothers don't have to do anything except to be there. They're old so they shouldn't play hard or run. It is enough if they take us to the market where the pretend horse is, and have a lot of pennies ready. Or if they take us for walks, they should slow down past things like pretty leaves and caterpillars. They should never say "hurry-up".

'Usually grandmothers are fat, but not too fat to tie your shoes. They wear glasses and funny underwear. They can take their teeth and gums off.

'Grandmothers don't have to be smart, only answer questions like, "Why isn't God married?" and "How come dogs chase cats?"

'Grandmothers don't talk baby-talk like visitors do, because it is hard to understand. When they read to us, they don't skip or mind if it is the same story over again.

'Everybody should try to have a grandmother, especially if you don't have television, because they are the only grown-ups who have time.'

*A nine-year-old*

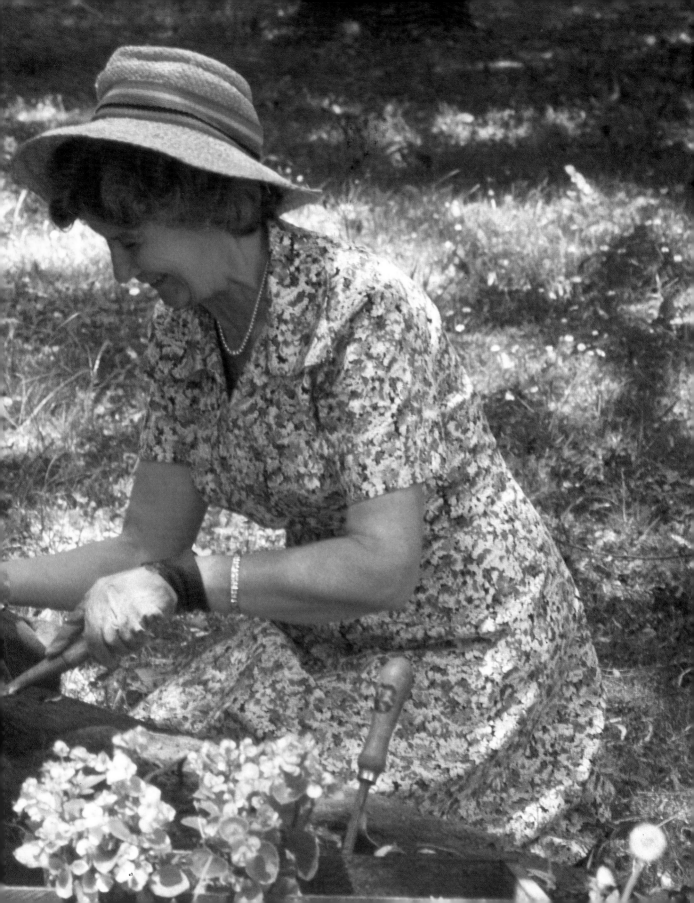

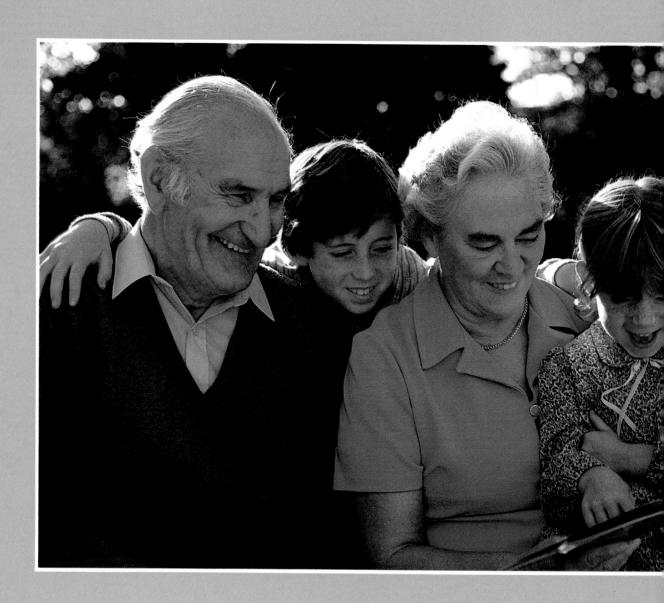

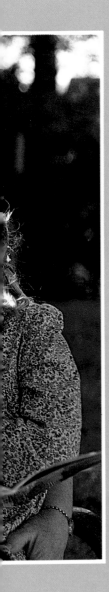

# THANK YOU

Thank you, God, for this time of my life. Thank you for the freedom to enjoy it. Thank you that the slackening of the demands of home life mean that I can enjoy being part of the working world once more. Thank you for the new friends and the fresh experiences that have come into my life because of it. I'm grateful, too, for the time that I can spend with my husband. We can actually talk now, without battling against crying babies, arguing children or transistor radios played at full volume. Thank you that we have still so many things to talk about!

Thank you, too, for grown-up children who are living their own lives and yet still want to be part of ours. For grandchildren who dance into our home and fill it with joy, but whose broken nights, tantrums and school problems are the main responsibility of someone else!

There are days, of course, on which I forget to be thankful. Occasions when I covet my daughter's fresh prettiness and the physical energy of younger friends. When I long for the fun of being at the centre of a growing family once again. Sometimes, God, you know that I do wish that I could turn the clock back, that I hanker after what might have been.

At those moments, remind me about the pressures as well as the privileges of being younger – and help me to be supportive and sympathetic to those who are experiencing them. And teach me to treasure the time that I have. Time to live and love and laugh. Time to learn more about myself, those around me and my God.

# MY FUTURE SELF

There was a time in my own life when I wondered about the value of growing and being old. No more. I do not want to miss my old age any more than I would choose to have skipped childhood or adolescence. But I do feel an increased sense of responsibility to this future self, and to all those whose lives may cross my path. What kind of old man will I be, given the chance? The answer to that question depends largely on the kind of person I am right now. For growing old is an ongoing project. . .through the lifespan.

*Robert Kastenbaum*


*You can't control the length of your life,*
*    but you can control its width and depth.*
*You can't control the contour of your countenance,*
*    but you can control its expression.*
*You can't control the other person's opportunities,*
*    but you can grasp your own. . .*
*Why worry about the things you can't control?*
*Get busy controlling things that depend on you.*

Myron J. Taylor


There's so much of me, in me, Lord.
I ask that as I get older
You won't let all the me in me solidify
So that you can't empty me of myself,
So that I am not pliable, usable, mouldable, shapable.
Because most of all, Lord,
I desire to be moulded by your hand,
    filled with your Spirit, used for your service.
That takes emptying – of me, and filling full of you.
Help me, Lord.

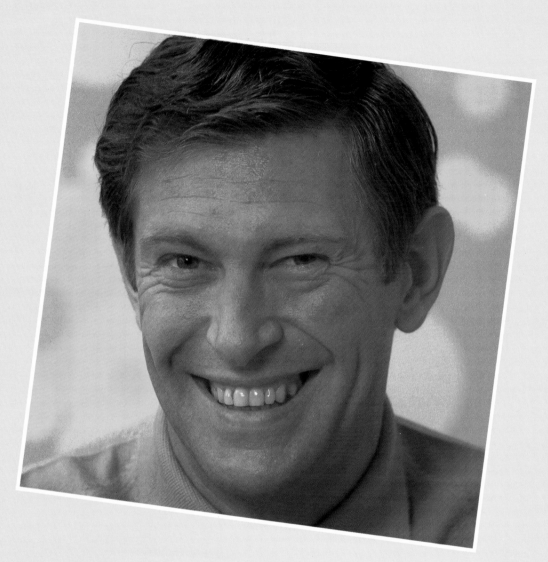

Lord, make old people tolerant,
Young folk sympathetic,
Great folk humble,
Busy folk patient,
Bad folk good,
And make me what I ought to be.

Anon

# TRUE GREATNESS

Try not to become a man of success, but a man
of value.

*Albert Einstein*

To be popular at home is a great achievement.
The man who is loved by the house cat, by the
dog, by the neighbour's children and by his
own wife, is a great man, even if he has never
had his name in *Who's Who*.

*Thomas Dreier*

It seemed as if everyone who was anyone
attended the ceremony in memory of you: civic
officials and business colleagues; strangers too
– men with letters after their names, who
valued your work. They came with kind words
of appreciation and support, taking the front
seats, anxious to see and to be seen.
   But today, five years on, who really
remembers? It is not the well-known but the
ordinary people – those whose lives you
touched with words of counsel, words of love
and words of faith and hope. Those to whom
you spoke of Jesus and challenged to commit
their lives to him. They are the living
memorials, the real and lasting tribute to a life
invested in others. This is an investment that
will survive time, and go on into eternity. An
investment which will receive the only accolade
that really matters: 'Well done, good and
faithful servant; enter into the joy of your Lord.'

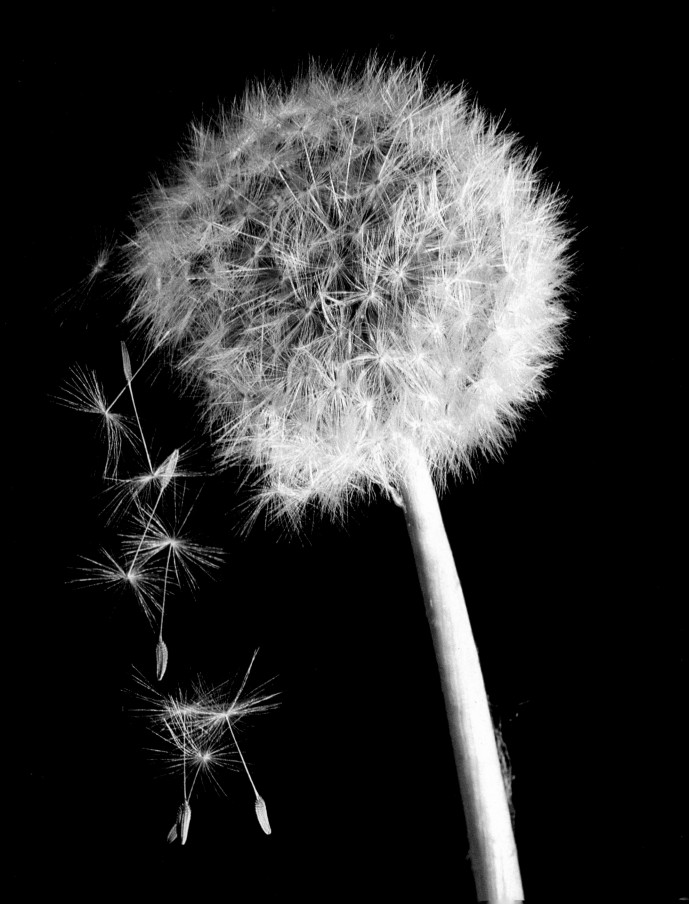

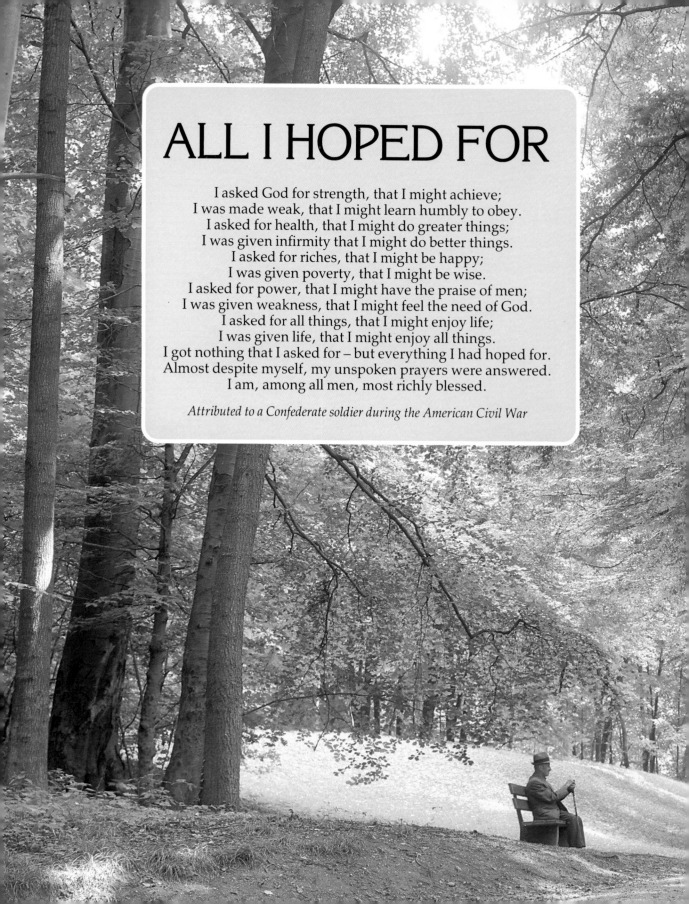

# ALL I HOPED FOR

I asked God for strength, that I might achieve;
I was made weak, that I might learn humbly to obey.
I asked for health, that I might do greater things;
I was given infirmity that I might do better things.
I asked for riches, that I might be happy;
I was given poverty, that I might be wise.
I asked for power, that I might have the praise of men;
I was given weakness, that I might feel the need of God.
I asked for all things, that I might enjoy life;
I was given life, that I might enjoy all things.
I got nothing that I asked for – but everything I had hoped for.
Almost despite myself, my unspoken prayers were answered.
I am, among all men, most richly blessed.

*Attributed to a Confederate soldier during the American Civil War*

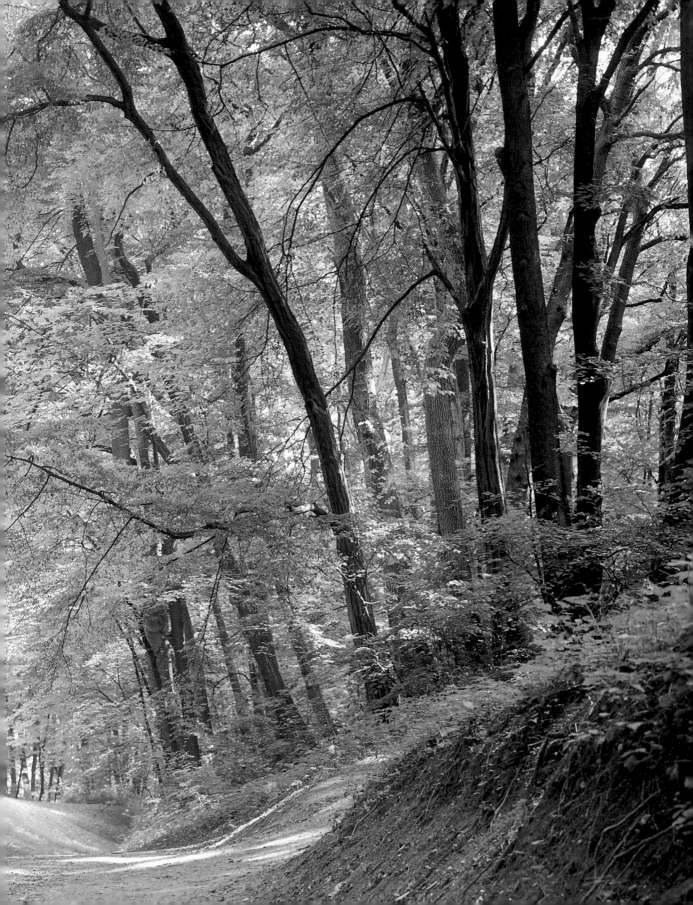

# THE LETTER

The letter lay, fragile and stained, on top of the pile. It was hard going through my mother's things. Missing her was still so new. I looked at the date. It had been written by a friend to my mother in 1939, shortly after my father died.

'Dear One,' it began, 'it hurts so terribly, doesn't it? Accept the pain if you can. Say, "Yes, because I have loved and now lost, I must cry for a while. I must hold this ache of loneliness within myself and say, this is the price I pay for having loved. I will accept this price and pay it in gratitude for the love I was blessed to know, for I would not have wanted to be without that love. I will pay this price, God, and I thank You for the wonderful years we shared."

'I think He must have cried on the day that His son hung dead on the cross, don't you think so? Don't you think that because He, too, is familiar with tears, dear friend, He is especially close to you right now?

'I weep with you, and my love surrounds you. Please write and let me know your plans, and if there is anything at all I can do to help.'

I folded the letter and slipped it back into the envelope, grateful for this healing message from the past.

*Doris Haase*

I would say to those who mourn, look on each day that comes as a challenge, as a test of courage. The pain will come in waves, some days worse than others, for no apparent reason. Accept the pain. Little by little you will find new strength, new vision, born of the very pain and loneliness which seem, at first, impossible to master.

*Daphne du Maurier*

*From tomorrow on*
*I shall be sad.*
*From tomorrow on –*
*not today.*
*Today I will be glad,*
*and every day*
*no matter how bitter it may be*
*I shall say*
*From tomorrow on I shall be sad,*
*not today.*

Written by a Jewish girl
in a concentration camp

# GUIDELINES

He gave us wise advice that day. . .

'We have to recognize,' he said, 'that all the major turning-points in our lives require a certain amount of forward planning – and retirement is no exception. We may dread it, ignore it until the day dawns, or anticipate it realistically and plan for it enthusiastically. In my experience, it is those who take the third course who seem to gain maximum enjoyment from these special years.

'Retirement dreams are, of course, as varied as the individuals who dream them, but even dreams have to be rooted in reality if they are to come true. So build your 'castle in the air' on a firm foundation, by taking the time *now* to ask yourself four key questions.

'Where shall I live?
Remember that a new area needs to be explored thoroughly and experienced at every season of the year. Fresh faces and fine views are not always an adequate substitute for old friends and familiarity.

'What shall I live on?
Less money does not necessarily spell less enjoyment, but it may mean that expensive items are not easily replaced. So it is both enjoyable and good sense to establish a "retirement chest", using sales and special offers to stock it, and to aim to start this new phase of life with as many belongings as possible in good repair.

'What shall I do?
We can look on retirement as the end of a working life, or a great opportunity to exchange one set of interests for others that we have always wanted to pursue. But hobbies, interests and friendships do not just happen – they have to be actively sought. And since a pleasure shared is a pleasure doubled, we might well aim to include things that we can do with others, as well as interests that we can enjoy alone.

'What shall I live for?
This is, perhaps, the most important question of all, for someone without a purpose for living is someone who merely exists. Jesus said, "Be concerned above everything else with the kingdom of God and what he requires of you, and he will provide you with all these other things." This is a motivation that has a transforming effect on any and every stage of life.'

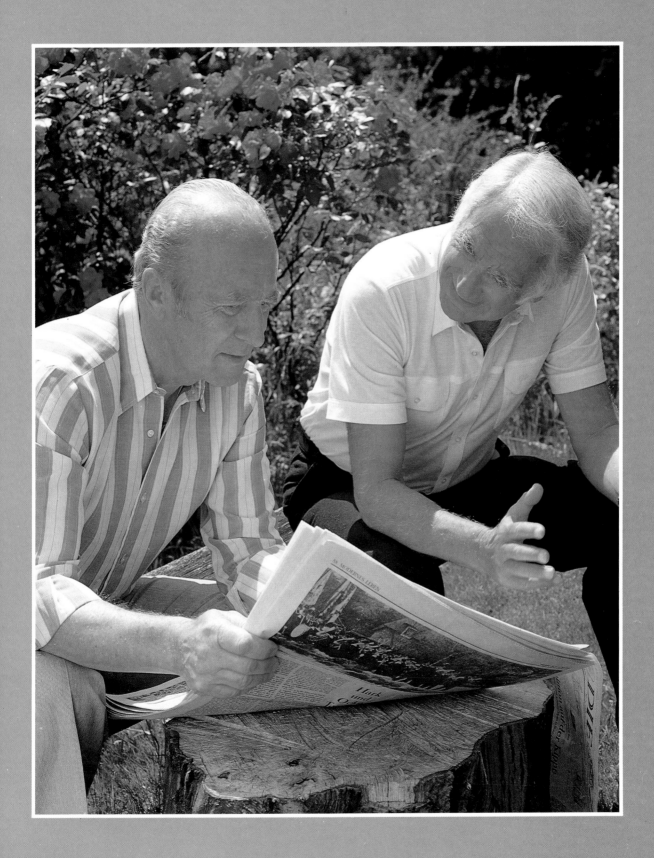

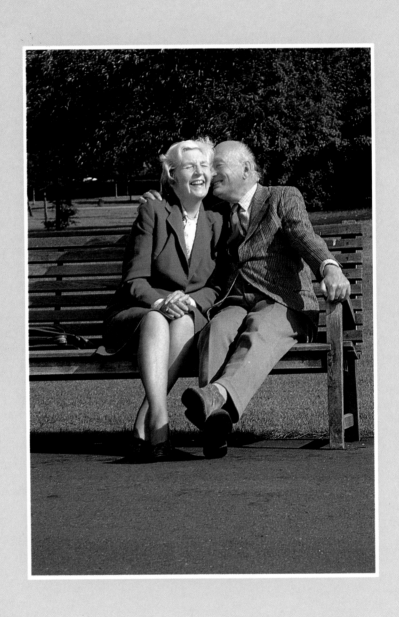

# LANDMARK

*The important thing at sixty is to remember we are not on the scrap-heap. There are great things we can still do.*

Robert Dougall

*Birthdays have always been special days, Lord. Days on which to look back, to look forward, to take stock and dream a little. Days to celebrate.*

*And yet I wondered, Lord, when I got up this morning. Could this day truly be a cause for celebrations, marking the beginning of a decade and the ending of her working life. How would she feel?*

*Of course, I should have known, Lord. Known that you would have something to say both to and through this long-time child of yours. A word to me and all of us who grasp your gift of years reluctantly.*

*My fears were foolishness. There were no ifs or buts to mar her day. With laughter she accepted our good wishes, then spoke enthusiastically of all that lies ahead.*

*'Today I reach the turning point of sixty! A landmark certainly,' she said, 'but one I reach with great excitement. Don't pity me. For I would not change places with a single one of you. Even if I could, I would not choose to be either one day older or a moment younger. My heavenly Father planned that I should reach this age at this time, while living in this place, for his good purpose. This day marks both an end and a beginning. The past I leave with him without regret and step out joyfully to meet the future he has planned.'*

*Every day and every hour is a new beginning with God. It makes no difference what the past has contained of failure or success, the present and the future are all with which we need be concerned.*

Donald Grey Barnhouse

*'It's not where you've been, it's where you're going that counts.'*

# KEEP ME YOUNG

I have been giving thought, Lord
   – you have a minute? – to getting old.
Natural enough as the years pass.

Getting old, a fellow said, is all in the mind.
True. It's also inclined to get into the joints,
   the digestion, and the poor old feet.
Spectacles appear, then a second pair.
Certain powers wane. Expected; allowed for.
But the fellow's right, or nearly right.

Now, Lord. To the point.
What if the mind gets stiff in the joints?
   Where are you then?
What if the mind goes lame, needs two pairs of specs?
Then, it would seem, a person's got trouble.
I mean, if the mind is in charge, and
   starts taking days off; loses grip.
   Where are you then?
Seems it's time for a person to shut the office.

So, Lord, please keep me young in the mind.
   Let me enjoy, Lord, let me enjoy.
If creaky I must be, and many-spectacled,
   and morning-stiff and food-careful,
If trembly-handed and slow-moving and
   breath-short and head-noddy,
I won't complain. Not a word.
If, with your help, dear Friend, there
   will dwell in this ancient monument,
A Young Mind. Please, Lord?

*David Kossoff*

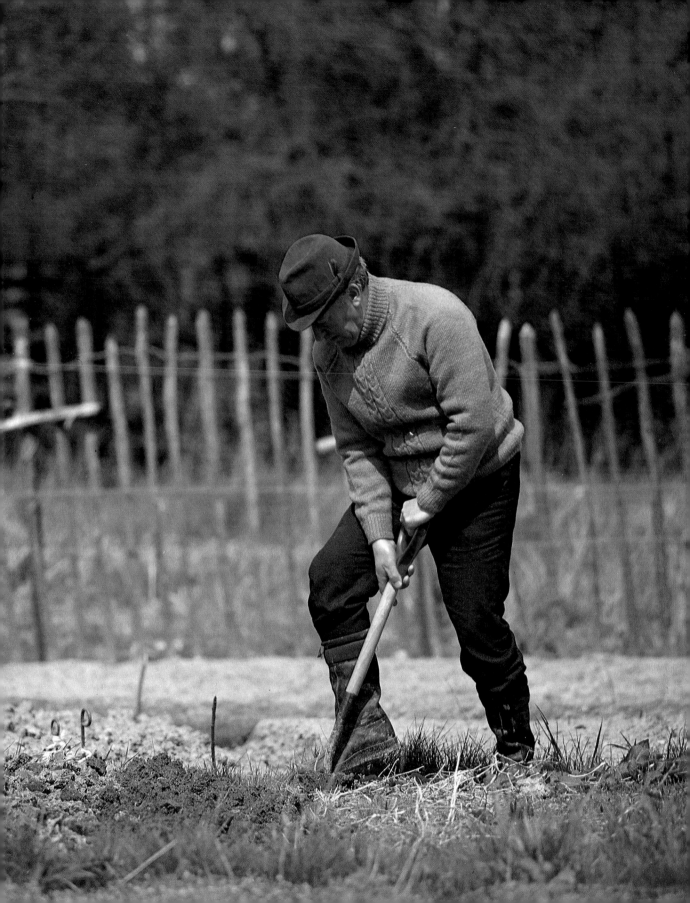

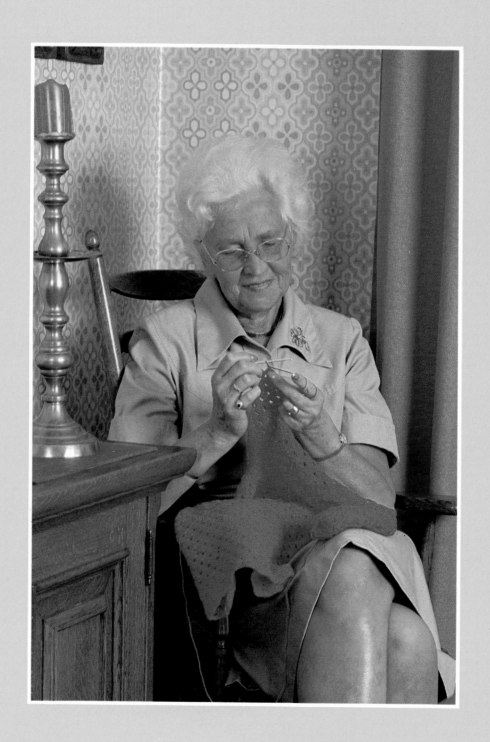

# ALL YOUR CARE

*Fear does not take away the grief of yesterday, nor does it solve the problems of tomorrow. All it does is rob you of the power of today.*

Corrie ten Boom


All of your care – tomorrow with its problems,
The lengthening shadows of the passing days,
The secret fears, of failure, weakness, suffering,
Of grief and loss, and straightened lonely ways,
   Leave it with Him, your future He will share,
   For you are His, the object of His care.

*Joan Suisted*


*'God has said,*
  *"Never will I leave you;*
   *never will I forsake you."*
*So we say with confidence,*
  *"The Lord is my helper; I will not be afraid." '*

The Book of Hebrews


The time comes to most of us when, whether we like it or not, old age and failing powers force us into solitude. Many people dread this time, and of course we cannot lapse into laziness and become an increasing burden to others. We must keep going while we can. But inevitably we shall become more and more alone.

If we have longed for solitude and learned to love it because we find God there, it should be that the last years of a long life will be the happiest of all, lived so close to Him, that His love and life can shine through us to countless souls.

*Margaret Evening*

# ON THE OTHER SIDE

'Jesus said. . ."I am the resurrection and the life. He who believes in me will live, even though he dies; and whoever lives and believes in me will never die." '

John's Gospel

Just as a good mariner, when he draws near to the harbour, lets down his sails and enters it gently with slight headway on; so we ought to let down the sails of our worldly pursuits and turn to God with all our heart, so that we may come to that haven with all composure, and with all peace. . .There is, in such a death, no pain nor any bitterness; but as a ripe apple lightly and without violence detaches itself from its bough, so our soul severs itself from the body where it has dwelt.

*Dante Alighieri*

There'll be no fear in heaven! 'He who sits on the throne will spread his tent over them'. That's a picture of heaven where all our fears will vanish in God's protecting presence.

There'll be no hunger or thirst. That's a picture of complete satisfaction which none of us can ever fully know on earth. But when we see Jesus face to face. . .there will be no inner cravings or emptiness.

There will be no suffering: 'The sun will not beat upon them, nor any scorching heat.' There will be no depressions, neuroses, anxieties, pressures, tensions, tiredness or old age.

There will be no loneliness: 'The Lamb at the centre of the throne will be their Shepherd; he will lead them to springs of living water'.

There will be no tears: 'God will wipe away every tear from their eyes'. Every cause of sadness will disappear in God's presence. We will be comforted beyond measure.

*David Watson*

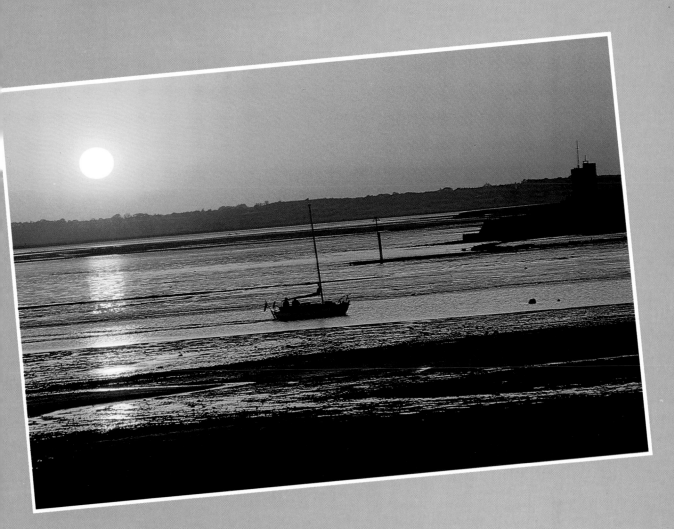

'My sword I give to him who shall succeed me in my pilgrimage and my courage and skill to him who can get it. My marks and scars I carry with me as a sign that I have fought His battles who will now be my rewarder.' So Mr Valiant for Truth passed over and all the trumpets sounded for him on the other side.

*John Bunyan*

'*"Death has been swallowed up in victory."*
  *"Where, O death, is your victory?*
    *Where, O death is your sting?"*
*The sting of death is sin. . .But thanks be to God!*
*He gives us the victory through our Lord Jesus Christ.'*

Paul: from the New Testament